The Ultimate Mediterranean Dinner Cookbook Recipes for Beginners

Vibrant Recipes for Everyday Home Cooking!

Hanna Briggs

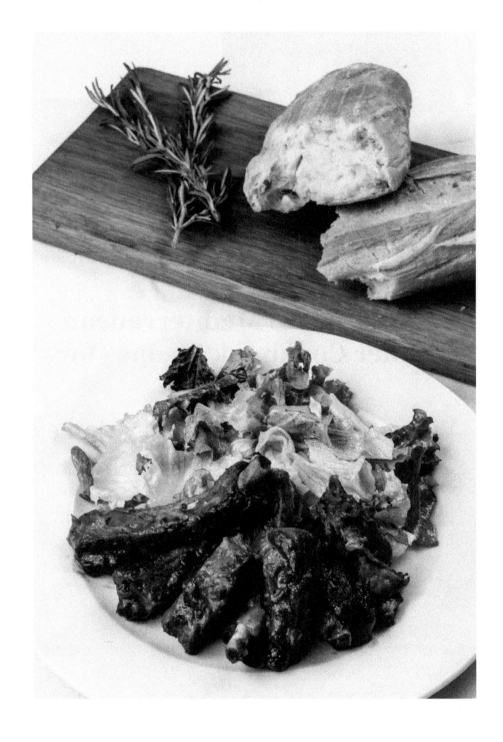

Table of contents

Introduction

Consuming the Mediterranean diet minimalizes the use of processed foods. It has been related to a reduced level of risk in developing numerous chronic diseases. It also enhances life expectancy. Several kinds of research have demonstrated many benefits in preventing cardiovascular disease, atrial fibrillation, breast cancer, and type 2 diabetes. Many pieces of evidence indicated a pattern that leads to low lipid, reduction in oxidative stress, platelet aggregation, and inflammation, and modification of growth factors and hormones involved in cancer.

Reduces Heart Diseases

According to research studies, the Mediterranean diet, which focuses on omega-3 ingredients and mono-saturated fats, reduces heart disease risk. It decreases the chances of cardiac death. The use of olive oil maintains the blood pressure levels. It is suitable for reducing hypertension. It also helps in combating the disease-promoting impacts of oxidation. This diet discourages the use of hydrogenated oils and saturated fats, which can cause heart disease.

Weight-loss

If you have been looking for diet plans for losing weight without feeling hungry, the Mediterranean diet can give you long term results. It is one of the best approaches. It is sustainable as it provides the most realistic approach to eat to feel full and energetic. This diet mostly consists of nutrient-dense food. It gives enough room for you to choose between low-carb and lower protein food. Olive oil consumed in this diet has antioxidants, natural vitamins, and some crucial fatty acids. It all improves your overall health. The Mediterranean diet focuses on natural foods, so there is very little room for junk and processed foods contributing to health-related issues and weight gain.

Most people trying the Mediterranean diet have gained positive results in cutting their weight. It is a useful option for someone looking forward to weight-loss as it provides the most unique and simple way to lose the overall calories without even changing your lifestyle that much. When you try to decrease calorie intake, losing weight is inevitable dramatically. But it will not benefit you. It will cause many health problems for you, including severe muscle loss. When you go for a Mediterranean diet, the body moves towards a sustainable model that burns calories slowly. So, it is crucial to practice the right approach and choose fat burning and more effective weight loss.

Prevents Cancer

The cornerstone of this diet is plant-based ingredients, especially vegetables and fruits. They help in preventing cancer. A plant-based diet provides antioxidants that help in protecting your DNA from damage and cell mutation. It also helps in lowering inflammation and delaying tumor growth. Various studies found that olive oil is a natural way to prevent cancer. It also decreases colon and bowel cancers. The plant-based diet balances blood sugar. It also sustains a healthy weight.

Prevents Diabetes

Numerous studies found that this healthy diet functions as an anti-inflammatory pattern, which helps fight the diseases related to chronic inflammation, Type 2 diabetes, and metabolic syndrome. It is considered very effective in preventing diabetes as it controls the insulin levels, which is a hormone to control the blood sugar levels and causes weight gain. Intake of a well-balanced diet consisting of fatty acids alongside some healthy carbohydrates and proteins is the best gift to your body. These foods help your body in burning fats more efficiently, which also provides energy. Due to the consumption of these kinds of foods, the insulin resistance level becomes non-existent, making it impossible to have high blood sugar.

Anti-aging

Choosing a Mediterranean diet without suffering from malnutrition is the most efficient and consistent anti-aging intervention. It undoubtedly expands lifespan, according to the research. The study found that the longevity biomarkers, i.e., body temperature and insulin level, and the DNA damage decreased significantly in humans by the Mediterranean diet. Other mechanisms also prove the claim made by researchers in explaining the anti-aging effects of adopting the Mediterranean diet, including reduced lipid peroxidation, high efficiency of oxidative repair, increased antioxidant defense system, and reduced mitochondrial generation rate.

Maintains Blood Sugar Level

The Mediterranean diet focuses on healthy carbs and whole grains. It has a lot of significant benefits. Consumption of whole-grain foods, like buckwheat, quinoa, and wheat berries instead of refined foods, helps you maintain blood sugar levels that ultimately gives you enough energy for the whole day.

Enhances Cognitive Health

The Mediterranean diet helps in preserving memory. It is one of the most useful steps for Alzheimer's treatment and dementia. Cognitive disorders occur when our brains do not get sufficient dopamine, which is a crucial chemical vital for mood regulation, thought processing, and body movements. Healthy fats like olive oil and nuts are good at fighting cognitive decline, mostly an age-related issue. They help counter some harmful impacts of the free radicals, inflammation, and toxins caused by having a low diet. The Mediterranean diet proves to be beneficial in decreasing

the risk of Alzheimer's to a great extent. Foods like yogurt help in having a healthy gut that improves mood, cognitive functioning, and memory.

Better Endurance Level

Mediterranean diet helps in fat loss and maintains muscle mass. It improves physical performance and enhances endurance levels. Research done on mice has shown positive results in these aspects. It also improves the health of our tissues in the long-term. The growth hormone also offers increased levels as a result of the Mediterranean diet. Which ultimately helps in improving metabolism and body composition.

Keeps You Agile

The nutrients from the Mediterranean diet reduces your risk of muscle weakness and frailty. It increases longevity. When your risk of heart disease reduces, it also reduces the risk of early death. It also strengthens your bones. Certain compounds found in olive oil help in preserving bone density. It helps increase the maturation and proliferation of the bone cells—dietary patterns of the Mediterranean diet help prevent osteoporosis.

Healthy Sleep Patterns

Our eating habits have a considerable impact on sleepiness and wakefulness. Some Mediterranean diet believers have reported an improved sleeping pattern as a result of changing their eating patterns. It has a considerable impact on your sleep because they regulate the circadian rhythm that determines our sleep patterns. If you have a regulated and balanced circadian rhythm, you will fall asleep quite quickly. You will also feel refreshed when you wake up. Another theory states that having the last meal will help you digest the food way before sleep. Digestion works best when you are upright.

Apart from focusing on plant-based eating, the Mediterranean diet philosophy emphasizes variety and moderation, living a life with perfect harmony with nature, valuing relationships in life, including sharing and enjoying meals, and having an entirely active lifestyle. The Mediterranean diet is at the crossroads. With the traditions and culture of three millennia, the Mediterranean diet lifestyle made its way to the medical world a long time ago. It has progressively recognized and became one of the successful and healthiest patterns that lead to a healthy lifestyle.

Besides metabolic, cardiovascular, cognitive, and many other benefits, this diet improves your life quality. Therefore, it is recommended today by many medical professionals worldwide. Efforts are being made in both non--Mediterranean and Mediterranean populations to make everyone benefit from the fantastic network of eating habits and patterns that began in old-time and which became a medical recommendation for a healthy lifestyle.

What to Eat and what to avoid

Fruits and vegetables: Mediterranean diet is one of the plant-based diet plans. Fresh fruits and vegetables contain a large number of vitamins, nutrients, fibers, minerals, and antioxidants

Fruits: Apple, berries, grapes, peaches, fig, grapefruit, dates, melon, oranges and pears.

Vegetables: Spinach, Brussels sprout, kale, tomatoes, kale, summer squash, onion, cauliflower, peppers, cucumbers, turnips, potatoes, sweet potatoes, and parsnips.

Seeds and nuts: Seeds and nuts are rich in monounsaturated fats and omega- 3 fatty acids.

Seeds: pumpkin seeds, flax seeds, sesame seeds, and sunflower seeds. Nuts: Almond, hazelnuts, pistachios, cashews, and walnuts.

Whole grains: Whole grains are high in fibers and they are not processed so they do not contain unhealthy fats like trans-fats compare to processed ones.

Whole grains: Wheat, quinoa, rice, barley, oats, rye, and brown rice. You can also use bread and pasta which is made from whole grains.

Fish and seafood: Fish are the rich source of omega-3 fatty acids and proteins. Eating fish at least once a week is recommended here. The healthiest way to consume fish is to grill it. Grilling fish taste good and never need extra oil.

Fish and seafood: salmon, trout, clams, mackerel, sardines, tuna and shrimp.

Legumes: Legumes (beans) are a rich source of protein, vitamins, and fibers. Regular consumption of beans helps to reduce the risk of diabetes, cancer and heart disease.

Legumes: Kidney beans, peas, chickpeas, black beans, fava beans, lentils, and pinto beans.

Spices and herbs: Spices and herbs are used to add the taste to your meal.

Spices and herbs: mint, thyme, garlic, basil, cinnamon, nutmeg, rosemary, oregano and more.

Healthy fats: Olive oil is the main fat used in the Mediterranean diet. It helps to reduce the risk of inflammatory disorder, diabetes, cancer, and heart- related disease. It also helps to increase HDL (good cholesterol) levels and decrease LDL (bad cholesterol) levels into your body. It also helps to lose weight.

Fats: Olive oil, avocado oil, walnut oil, extra virgin olive oil, avocado, and olives.

Dairy: Moderate amounts of dairy products are allowed during the Mediterranean diet. The dairy product contains high amounts of fats.

Dairy: Greek yogurt, skim milk and cheese.

Food to avoid

Refined grains: Refined grains are not allowed in a Mediterranean diet. It raises your blood sugar level. Refined grains like white bread, white rice, and pasta.

Refined oils: Oils like vegetable oils, cottonseed oils, and soybean oils are completely avoided from the Mediterranean diet. It raises your LDL (bad cholesterol) level.

Added Sugar: Added sugar is not allowed in the Mediterranean diet. These types of artificial sugars are found in table sugar, soda, chocolate, ice cream, and candies. It raises your blood sugar level.

You should consume only natural sugars in the Mediterranean diet.

Processed foods: Generally Processed foods come in boxes. Its low-fat food should not be eaten during the diet. It contains a high amount of trans-fats. Mediterranean diet is all about to eat fresh and natural food.

Trans-fat and saturated fats: In this category of food contains butter and margarine.

Processed Meat: Mediterranean diet does not allow to use of processed meat such as bacon, hot dogs and sausage.

21 days meal plan with meal prep tips
Meal Preparation tips

Use extra-virgin olive oil instead of butter

Butter contains saturated fats. Saturated fats are not recommended during the Mediterranean diet. Instead of butter, you can use extra virgin olive oil. Olive oil is heart-healthy oil contains good fat like polyunsaturated and monounsaturated fats. You can also use olive oil over salad for dressing. Extra virgin olive oil is healthy fat recommended in the Mediterranean diet.

Add more avocados into your diet

Avocados contains healthy monounsaturated fats which is one of the good fats recommended in the Mediterranean diet.

Add whole grain and brown rice

Mediterranean diet recommends brown rice and whole grains in the diet because grains are the best source of protein and they are rich in fibers. The bowl of oatmeal is one of the perfect breakfasts during the cold season.

Eat more legumes

Legumes are full of nutrients they are rich in fibers, high in proteins and low in fats. Legumes are also your budget-friendly food. It includes lentils, chickpeas, dried peas, and beans.

Consume plenty of fruits

Fruits are an essential part of the Mediterranean diet. Fruits are a good source of vitamins, fibers, and antioxidants. It is the best source of natural sugar and it is available easily. It helps to fulfill your sugar carving.

Don't overdo alcohol

Alcohol is part of the Mediterranean lifestyle. One of the misunderstandings is about alcohol is that you can drink lots of alcohol in the form of red wine. A moderate amount of alcohol is allowed while eating a meal.

Eat more fish

Fish is the best source of protein and omega-3 fatty acids. Specially eat fatty fish like mackerel, salmon, and sardines. One of the best ways to eat fish is to grill it. Grilled fish has great taste and never take extra oil for cooking.

Focus on the meal

While eating your meal you must concentrate on your meat. Always eat your meal slowly, give yourself 20 minutes to eat a meal. Stop eating your food in front of the television. You must focus and concentrate on your meal while eating.

Grocery list for each day

Now that you have begun taking steps towards integrating the Mediterranean diet into your lifestyle, the time has come to go shopping. Stocking your refrigerator and pantry with the right ingredients will go a long way to ensuring your success on this easy diet.

To make things easier for you and because I like to categorize, I've made a shopping list that will cover almost all your cooking needs:

Protein

Unsalted nuts

Fish and shellfish

Beans, peas, and lentils

Lean meats

Skinless chicken and poultry where possible

Poultry

Eggs

Dairy

All dairy should either be low-fat or fat-free.

Yogurt Sour cream

Almond milk Rice milk Hemp milk Soy milk

Cheese (try to find the reduced fat cheeses)

Spices

Salt Pepper Cinnamon Cumin

Chili powder Cayenne pepper Curry powder

Honey Vinegar Garlic Ginger Herbs

Whole grains

Brown rice Quinoa

Whole grain bread Whole wheat pasta

Whole wheat flour, preferably stone milled Whole grain couscous

Vegetables

Fruit

Any fresh vegetables. Do try to incorporate a lot of dark leafy greens in your diet since they are full of antioxidants and other nutrients.

Frozen vegetables

Any fresh fruit that you enjoy. Aim to have seasonal fruits. This will help keep your budget cost-effective while you enjoy fresh produce.

Frozen fruit

Seeds Oatmeal Chickpeas Black beans

White beans

Low-sodium broth Other necessities

Dry red wine such as cabernet sauvignon Dark chocolate, roughly around the 70% mark Unsweetened cocoa

21 meal plan

Day 1

Breakfast: Italian Basil and Mushroom Omelet

Lunch: Provençal Vegetable Soup

Dinner: Steamed Italian Halibut with Green Grapes

Snacks: Tender Roasted Sweet Potatoes with Savory Tahini Sauce

Day 2

Breakfast: Mediterranean Fruit Oatmeal

Lunch: Grilled Chicken Salad with Fennel, Orange, and Raisins

Dinner: Hearty Root Veggie and Beef Stew

Snacks: Homemade Whole Wheat Pita Bread

Day 3

Breakfast: Smoked Salmon and Asparagus Omelet

Lunch: Simple Rosemary Shrimp Polenta

Dinner: Italian Chicken Stew with Potatoes, Bell Peppers and Tomatoes

Snacks: Crisp Spiced Cauliflower with Feta Cheese

Day 4

Breakfast: Mediterranean Muesli

Lunch: Tunisian Turnovers with Tuna, Egg and Tomato

Dinner: Eggplants with Tomato and Minced Lamb Stuffing

Snacks: Pumpkin Kibbeh

Day 5

Breakfast: Buckwheat Berry Crepes with Cottage Cheese

Lunch: Fish and Spinach Gratin

Dinner: Savory Roasted Sea Bass

Snacks: Oven Roasted Carrots with Olives and Cumin Yogurt Sauce

Day 6

Breakfast: No-Crust Broccoli and Cheese Quiche

Lunch: Calamari with Herb and Rice Stuffing

Dinner: Pork Roast with Zest Fig and Acorn Squash

Snacks: Bravas Potatoes with Roasted Tomato Sauce

Day 7

Breakfast: Banana-Strawberry Breakfast Smoothie

Lunch: Classic Niçoise Chicken

Dinner: Warm-Spiced Lamb Meatballs in Tomato Sauce

Snacks: Spring Peas and Beans with Zesty Thyme Yogurt Sauce

Day 8

Breakfast: Italian Basil and Mushroom Omelet

Lunch: Provençal Vegetable Soup

Dinner: Steamed Italian Halibut with Green Grapes

Snacks: Tender Roasted Sweet Potatoes with Savory Tahini Sauce

Day 9

Breakfast: Mediterranean Fruit Oatmeal

Lunch: Grilled Chicken Salad with Fennel, Orange, and Raisins

Dinner: Hearty Root Veggie and Beef Stew

Snacks: Homemade Whole Wheat Pita Bread

Day 10

Breakfast: Smoked Salmon and Asparagus Omelet

Lunch: Simple Rosemary Shrimp Polenta

Dinner: Italian Chicken Stew with Potatoes, Bell Peppers and Tomatoes

Snacks: Crisp Spiced Cauliflower with Feta Cheese

Day 11

Breakfast: Mediterranean Muesli

Lunch: Tunisian Turnovers with Tuna, Egg and Tomato

Dinner: Eggplants with Tomato and Minced Lamb Stuffing

Snacks: Pumpkin Kibbeh

Day 12

Breakfast: Buckwheat Berry Crepes with Cottage Cheese

Lunch: Fish and Spinach Gratin

Dinner: Savory Roasted Sea Bass

Snacks: Oven Roasted Carrots with Olives and Cumin Yogurt Sauce

Day 13

Breakfast: No-Crust Broccoli and Cheese Quiche

Lunch: Calamari with Herb and Rice Stuffing

Dinner: Pork Roast with Zest Fig and Acorn Squash

Snacks: Bravas Potatoes with Roasted Tomato Sauce

Day 14

Breakfast: Banana-Strawberry Breakfast Smoothie

Lunch: Classic Niçoise Chicken

Dinner: Warm-Spiced Lamb Meatballs in Tomato Sauce

Snacks: Spring Peas and Beans with Zesty Thyme Yogurt Sauce

Day 15

Breakfast: Italian Basil and Mushroom Omelet

Lunch: Provençal Vegetable Soup

Dinner: Steamed Italian Halibut with Green Grapes

Snacks: Tender Roasted Sweet Potatoes with Savory Tahini Sauce

Day 16

Breakfast: Mediterranean Fruit Oatmeal

Lunch: Grilled Chicken Salad with Fennel, Orange, and Raisins

Dinner: Hearty Root Veggie and Beef Stew

Snacks: Homemade Whole Wheat Pita Bread

Day 17

Breakfast: Smoked Salmon and Asparagus Omelet

Lunch: Simple Rosemary Shrimp Polenta

Dinner: Italian Chicken Stew with Potatoes, Bell Peppers and Tomatoes

Snacks: Crisp Spiced Cauliflower with Feta Cheese

Day 18

Breakfast: Mediterranean Muesli

Lunch: Tunisian Turnovers with Tuna, Egg and Tomato

Dinner: Eggplants with Tomato and Minced Lamb Stuffing

Snacks: Pumpkin Kibbeh

Day 19

Breakfast: Buckwheat Berry Crepes with Cottage Cheese

Lunch: Fish and Spinach Gratin

Dinner: Savory Roasted Sea Bass

Snacks: Oven Roasted Carrots with Olives and Cumin Yogurt Sauce

Day 20

Breakfast: No-Crust Broccoli and Cheese Quiche

Lunch: Calamari with Herb and Rice Stuffing

Dinner: Pork Roast with Zest Fig and Acorn Squash

Snacks: Bravas Potatoes with Roasted Tomato Sauce

Day 21

Breakfast: Banana-Strawberry Breakfast Smoothie

Lunch: Classic Niçoise Chicken

Dinner: Warm-Spiced Lamb Meatballs in Tomato Sauce

Snacks: Spring Peas and Beans with Zesty Thyme Yogurt Sauce

Mediterranean Diet Dinner Recipes

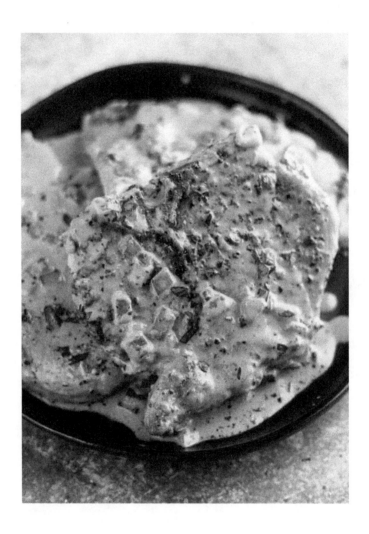

Vegetarian Lasagna
Servings: 6

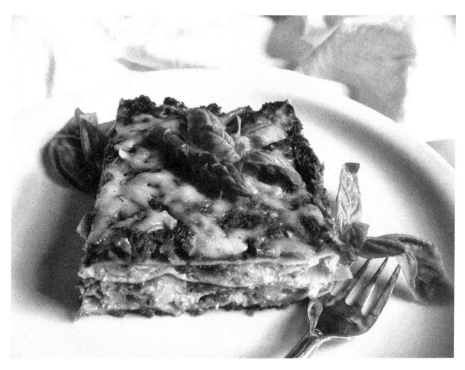

Ingredients:

- Sweet Onion, Sliced Thick
- 1 Eggplant, Sliced Thick
- Zucchini, Sliced Lengthwise Tablespoons Olive Oil
- 28 Ounces Canned tomatoes, Diced & Sodium Free
- 1 Cup Quartered, Canned & Water Packed Artichokes, Drained
- 2 Teaspoons Basil, Fresh & Chopped
- 2 Teaspoons Garlic, Minced
- 2 Teaspoons Oregano, Fresh & Chopped
- 12 Lasagna Noodles, Whole Grain & No Boil
- ¼ Teaspoon Red Pepper Flakes
- ¾ Cup Asiago Cheese, Grated

Directions:

1.   Start by heating your oven to 400, and then get out a baking sheet. Line it with foil before placing it to the side.

2.   Get out a large bowl and toss your zucchini, yellow squash, eggplant, onion and olive oil, making sure it's coated well.

3.   Arrange your vegetables on the baking sheet, roasting for twenty minutes. They should be lightly caramelized and tender.

4.   Chop your roasted vegetables before placing them in a bowl.

5.   Stir in your garlic, basil, oregano, artichoke hearts, tomatoes and red pepper flakes, spooning a quarter of this mixture in the bottom of a nine by thirteen baking dish. Arrange four lasagna noodles over this sauce, and continue by alternating it. Sprinkle with asiago cheese on top, baking for a half hour.

6.   Allow it to cool for fifteen minutes before slicing to serve.

Chili Calamari
Servings: 4

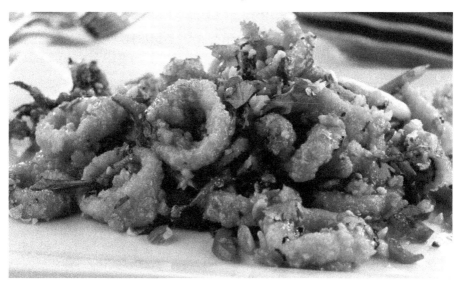

Ingredients:

- Lime, Juiced & Zested Tablespoons Olive Oil
- 1 Teaspoon Chili Powder
- ½ Teaspoon Cumin, Ground
- ¼ Teaspoon Sea Salt, Fine
- ¼ Teaspoon Black Pepper
- Tablespoons Cilantro, Fresh & Chopped
- 2 Tablespoons Red Bell Pepper, Minced
- 1 ½ lbs. Squid, Cleaned, Split Open & Cut into ½ Inch Rounds

Directions:

1.   Get out a bowl and mix your chili powder, cumin, lime juice, lime zest, olive oil, salt and pepper together. Add in your squid, and make sure it's well coated. Cover and allow it to marinate in the fridge for an hour.

2.   Preheat your oven to a broil and get out a baking sheet. Lay your squid on your baking sheet, broiling for eight minutes. You'll need to turn once in this time, and it should be tender.

3.   Garnish with red bell pepper and cilantro before serving.

Trout & Greens
Servings: 4

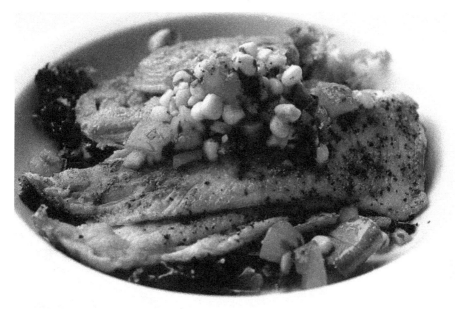

Ingredients:

- 2 Teaspoons Olive Oil + More for Greasing
- 2 Cups Swiss Chard, Chopped
- 2 Cups Kale, Chopped
- ½ Sweet Onion, Sliced Thin
- 4 Trout Fillets, Skin On & 5 Ounces Each Lemon, Zested
- ¼ Teaspoon Sea Salt, Fine
- ¼ Teaspoon Black Pepper

Directions:

1.   Start by heating your oven to 375, and then grease a nine by thirteen-inch baking dish using olive oil. Arrange your swiss chard, kale and onion on the bottom.

2.   Top with greens and then place your fish on top. Make sure the skin side is up, and drizzle with lemon juice and olive oil.

Season with salt and pepper before baking for fifteen minutes.
Serve with lemon zest.

Tuscan Chicken with Rice
Servings: 6

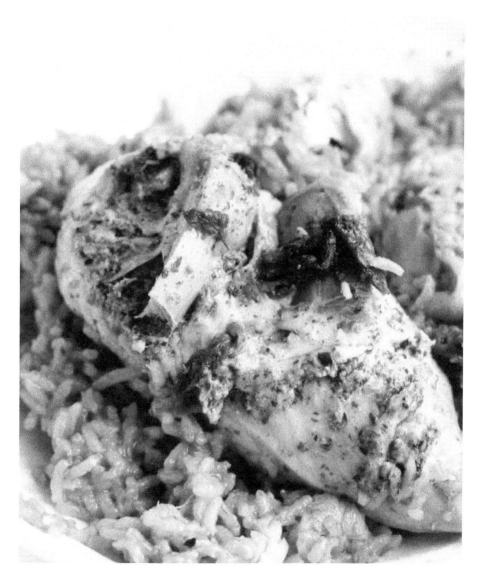

Ingredients:

- ¾ Cup Brown Rice
- Cup Cherry Tomatoes, Halved Yellow Bell Pepper, Diced

- ½ Red Onion, Chopped
- ¼ Cup Kalamata Olives, Sliced
- 4 Chicken Breasts, 4 Ounces Each, Boneless, Skinless, & Cut into 3 Pieces
- Teaspoons Oregano, Fresh & Chopped
- 1 Teaspoon Garlic Powder
- ½ Cup Goat Cheese,
- Crumbled Cups
- Chicken Stock, Sodium Free
- ½ Lemon, Juiced
- 1 Tablespoon Parsley, Fresh & Chopped

Directions:

1.　Start by heating your oven to 350, and then get out a bowl. Mix together your cherry tomatoes, red onion, bell pepper, olive sand brown rice. Spoon this mxi into a nine by thirteen-inch baking dish.

2.　Lay your chicken on top, and then season with garlic powder and oregano. Pour the lemon juice and chicken stock in.

3.　Cover and bake for forty to forty-five minutes. The rice should be cooked as well as the chicken. Fluff before serving with goat cheese and parsley.

Pork Chops & Peaches
Servings: 4

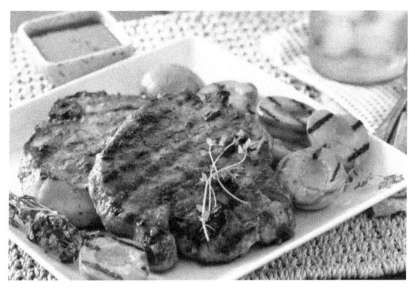

Ingredients:

- ½ Fennel Bulb, Chopped in 1 Inch Chunks
- 4 Pork Chops, Boneless,
- 5 Ounces Each & Trimmed
- 2 Tablespoons Olive Oil, Divided + More for Greasing
- 2 Peaches, Pitted & Quartered
- Sweet Onion, Peeled & Sliced Thin Tablespoons Balsamic Vinegar Teaspoon Thyme, Fresh & Chopped
- 1/4 Teaspoon Sea Salt, Fine
- ¼ Teaspoon Black Pepper

Directions:

1.   Heat your oven to 400, and then get out a nine by thirteen-inch baking dish. Make sure to grease it with olive oil before placing it to the side. Season your pork chops with salt and pepper.

2.   Get out a bowl and toss your onion, peaches, fennel, thyme,

balsamic vinegar, a tablespoon of olive oil and thyme. Roast them in your baking dish for twenty minutes.

3.   Get out a skillet, placing it over medium-high heat, and heat up your remaining oil.

4.   Add in your pork chops, searing for two minutes per side.

5.   Take your vegetables out of the oven and stir them. Place the pork chops on top, and then roast for another ten minutes. Your pork should be cooked all the way through.

Melitzanes Imam
Servings: 2

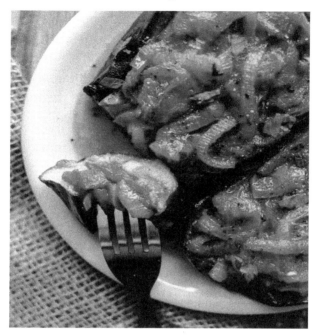

Ingredients:

- Eggplant
- Medium Chopped Onion
- 14.5-ounce can of Diced Tomatoes (Drained)
- 1 tablespoon of Minced Garlic
- 2 tablespoons of Olive Oil
- 1 teaspoon of Ground Cinnamon Pepper
- Salt

Directions:

1.   Preheat your oven to 350 degrees.

2.   Slice your eggplant in half lengthwise and hollow out both halves, leaving a 1-centimeter shell. Set the inside flesh to the side for later use. Place your shells on a baking tray. Drizzle with olive oil.

3.   Bake approximately 30 minutes until soft.

4.   Chop your leftover eggplant into small sized pieces. Heat 2 tablespoons of olive oil over a medium heat in a large skillet. Add your garlic and onion. Cook for 2 to 3 minutes, stirring often. Add your chopped eggplant and continue to cook until tender. Mix in your tomato paste and tomatoes until well blended. Simmer over a low heat until the eggplant halves baking in the oven are ready.

5.   Remove your eggplant shells from the oven and spoon in your eggplant and tomato mixture. Sprinkle some cinnamon over the top of each one.

6.   Place back in the oven and continue to cook for approximately 30 more minutes.

7.   Serve and Enjoy!

Greek Chicken Stew
Servings: 8

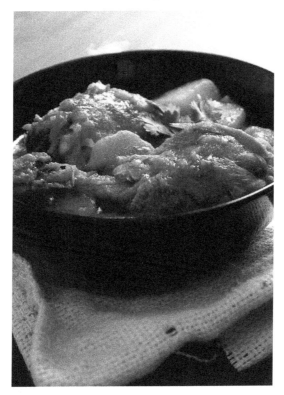

Ingredients

- 4 pound Whole Chicken (Cut Into Pieces)
- 1 cup of Olive Oil
- 10 Peeled Small Shallots teaspoons of Butte
- cloves of Finely Chopped Garlic
- 1 cup of Tomato Sauce
- 1/2 cup of Red Wine
- 2 tablespoons of Chopped Fresh Parsley
- 2 Bay Leaves
- 1/2 cups of Chicken Stock
- Pinch of Dried Oregano

- Ground Black Pepper
- Salt

Directions:

1.   Bring a big skillet of water to a boil. Add your shallots and cook for 3 minutes, uncovered, until tender. Drain in your colander and immediately immerse in ice water. Rinse with cold water for a few minutes until shallots are cold. This is done to halt the cooking process. When your shallots are cold, drain and set to the side.

2.   Heat your butter and olive oil in a large skillet over a medium heat until the butter is bubbling and melted. Add shallots and chicken pieces to your skillet and cook, turning over the chicken pieces until they are no longer pink on the inside and the shallots have turned translucent and softened. Should take about 15 minutes. Stir in your chopped garlic and cook approximately 3 minutes.

3.   Pour in your tomato sauce and red wine. Add the salt, pepper, bay leaves, oregano, and parsley. Pour your chicken stock over the chicken pieces to cover. Stir together well to combine.

4.   Simmer your stew, covered, over a medium-low heat for approximately 50 minutes.

5.   Serve and Enjoy!

Parma Wrapped Chicken w/ Mediterranean Vegetables
Servings: 2

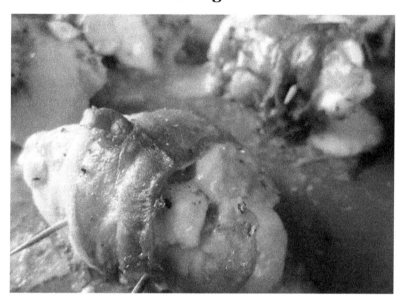

Ingredients

- 25-ounce Skinless Boneless Chicken Breast Halves
- 12 Cherry Tomatoes
- 4 0.5-ounce slices of Prosciutto Di Parma
- 1/2 pound of Baby red Potatoes (Cut Into Half)
- Red Onion (Cut Into 1/2 Inch Thick Wedges)
- 1 Zucchini (Halved Lengthwise & Cut Into 1 Inch Slices)
- Red Bell Peppers (Cut Into 1 Inch Pieces)
- tablespoons of Minced Garlic
- 1/4 teaspoon of Crushed Red Pepper Flakes
- 2 tablespoons of Olive Oil
- 1/2 teaspoon of Dried Thyme Leaves
- Ground Pepper

- Salt
- Toothpicks

Directions

1. Preheat your oven to 400 degrees.

2. Mix your zucchini, potatoes, tomatoes, and bell peppers in a big bowl. Add your thyme, garlic, and red pepper flakes. Toss your vegetable mix and season with your pepper and salt. Pour your olive oil over the veggies and toss to coat. Pour into your glass baking dish and bake in the oven for approximately 15 minutes.

3. Season chicken with pepper and salt. Wrap each of your chicken breasts with 2 slices of prosciutto and secure the prosciutto with a toothpick. Place on top of your vegetables and continue to bake for approximately 30 minutes until the chicken is no longer pink in the center.

4. Remove chicken from the baking dish for 5 minutes to cool. Divide your roasted vegetables among two plates. Remove the toothpicks from the chicken. Cut each piece of chicken into 5 diagonal slices. Fan your chicken out on top of your vegetables.

5. Serve and Enjoy!

Garlic-Braised Chicken w/ Olives and Mushrooms
Servings: 4

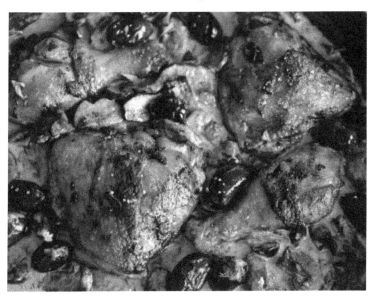

Ingredients

- Small Chicken (Cut Into Pieces)
- 1 tablespoon + 1 teaspoon of Olive Oil
- 16 cloves of Peeled & Smashed Garlic
- 10 ounces of Cremini Mushrooms (Trimmed & Halved)
- 1/2 cup of Pitted Green Olives
- 1/2 cup of White Wine
- 1/3 cup of Chicken Stock Coarse Salt
- Ground Pepper

Directions:

1.   Heat a large-sized skillet over a medium-high heat. Season chicken with pepper and salt. Add 1 tablespoon of your oil to the pan and swirl. Add your chicken, skin side down. Cook for 5 to 6

minutes until browned. Remove chicken from the pan. Set to the side.

2.   Add a teaspoon of oil to your pan. Add in your garlic and mushrooms. Cook for 5 to 6 minutes, stirring occasionally until they brown.

3.   Add your wine to the garlic and mushrooms. Bring to a boil and cook approximately 1 minute. Return your chicken to the pan.

4.   Add your chicken stock and olives to the pan. Bring water to a boil, then reduce the heat. Cover and simmer for 15 to 20 minutes until the chicken is cooked through.

5.   Serve and Enjoy!

Paprika Chicken Thighs w/ Brussels Sprouts
Servings: 4

Ingredients

- 4 Large Chicken Thighs (Skin Removed)
- pound of Brussels Sprouts (Trimmed & Halved)
- 1 Sliced Lemon
- 4 Small Quartered Shallots
- 1 teaspoon of Dried Thyme
- tablespoon of Smoked Paprika (Hot or Sweet) cloves of Minced Garlic
- 3/4 teaspoon of Salt
- tablespoons of Extra-Virgin Olive Oil
- 1/2 teaspoon of Ground Pepper

Directions:

1.   Position your rack in the lower third of your oven. Preheat the oven to 450 degrees.

2.   Combine your shallots, brussels sprouts, lemon, 2 tablespoons of oil and 1/4 teaspoon each of pepper and salt on a rimmed baking sheet.

3.   Mash your garlic and the remaining 1/2 teaspoon of salt to form a paste. Combine your paste with the thyme, paprika, remaining 1/4 teaspoon of pepper and 1 tablespoon of oil in a small-sized bowl. Rub your paste all over your chicken. Place your chicken into the brussels sprouts.

4.   Roast your chicken for 20 to 25 minutes in the oven until the brussels sprouts are tender and the thickest part of your chicken registers 165 degrees using a food thermometer. Remove from the oven.

5.   Serve and Enjoy!

Ziti With Olives and Sun-Dried Tomatoes
Servings: 6

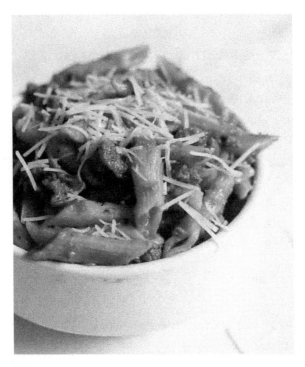

Ingredients

- 16-ounce package of Ziti Pasta
- 1/3 cup of Pitted & Sliced Black Greek Olives
- 2 Diced Anchovy Fillets
- 1/3 cup of Chopped Sun-Dried Tomatoes
- 2   teaspoons of Minced Garlic
- 2 tablespoons of Olive Oil
- 1/4 cup of Chopped Parsley Salt

Directions:

1.   Cook your pasta in a large skillet of boiling salted water until al dente.

2.   Meanwhile, place your sun-dried tomatoes, parsley, olives, anchovy fillets, garlic, and olive oil in a big serving bowl.

3.   Drain your pasta. Transfer to the serving bowl. Toss with your tomato mixture.

4.   Serve and Enjoy!

Mediterranean Fried Rice
Servings: 4

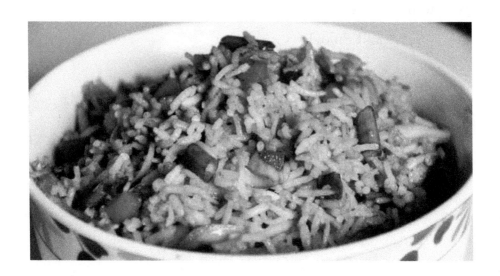

Ingredients:

- 1/2 cups of Cooked Rice

- 1 clove of Minced Garlic

- 2 tablespoons of Olive Oil

- 10-ounce package of Chopped Spinach (Drained & Thawed)

- 1/2 cup of Crumbled Feta Cheese w/ Herbs

- 4-ounce jar of Roasted Red Peppers (Drained & Chopped)

- 6- ounce jar of Marinated Artichoke Hearts (Drained & Quartered)

Directions:

1.   Heat your olive oil over a medium heat in a skillet. Add your garlic and cook for approximately 2 minutes until fragrant and starting to brown. Stir in your rice and cook for another 2 minutes, stirring often. Add your spinach and cook for 3 minutes until heated through.

2.   Stir your roasted red peppers and artichoke hearts into your rice mixture and cook for 2 minutes. Mix in your feta cheese. Remove from the heat.

3.   Serve and Enjoy!

Garlic Linguine
Servings: 4

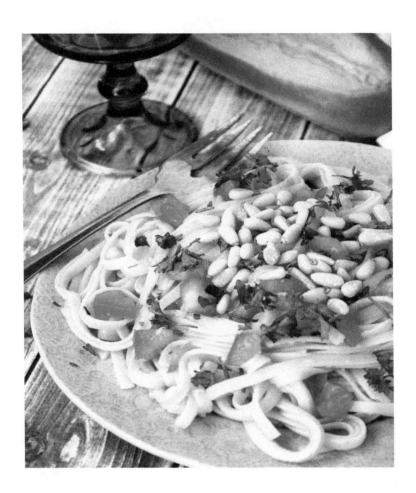

Ingredients

- 8-ounce package of Linguini Pasta
- 1 tablespoon of Minced Garlic
- 3 tablespoons of Olive Oil

- 1 tablespoon of Dried Oregano cups of Chopped Tomatoes
- 1 teaspoon of Dried Thyme
- 1 tablespoon of Dried Basil

Directions:

1. Cook your pasta in a big skillet of water until done. Drain pasta.

2. Heat oil in a saucepan. Add your garlic and cook for approximately 2 minutes, stirring often. Crush your herbs and add to your garlic.

3. Add your pasta. Heat through, stirring constantly. Fold in your tomatoes.

4. Serve and Enjoy!

Old-Fashioned Spaghetti & Meatballs
Servings: 6

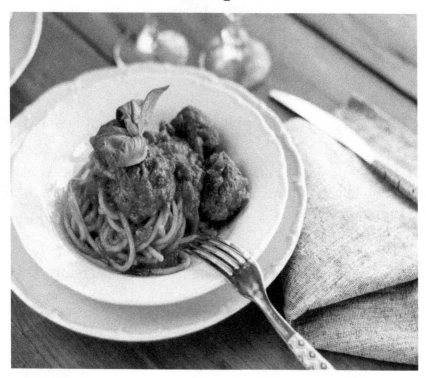

Ingredients

- Meatballs
- 4 ounces of Lean Ground Beef
- 1/3 cup of Bulgur
- 4 ounces of Hot Italian Sausage
- 1/2 cup of Hot Water
- Medium Finely Chopped Onion
- 2 cloves of Finely Chopped Garlic Large
- Egg Whites (Lightly Beaten)
- 1/2 teaspoon of Salt
- teaspoon of Dried Oregano cup of Fresh Breadcrumbs
- 1/2 teaspoon of Freshly Ground Pepper Sauce & Spaghetti
- 1 pound of Whole Wheat Spaghetti

- 3 cups of Prepared Marinara Sauce
- 1/2 cup of Freshly Grated Parmesan Cheese
- 1/2 cup of Chopped Fresh Parsley

Directions:

1. Combine your water and bulgur in a small-sized bowl. Allow to

stand until your bulgur is tender and all the liquid is absorbed. Should take about 30 minutes.

2. Preheat your oven to 350 degrees. Coat your rack with cooking spray and place it over your foil lined baking sheet.

3. Combine your sausage, ground beef, egg whites, oregano, onion, pepper, breadcrumbs, salt and your soaked bulgur in a big bowl. Mix together well. Form your mixture into 1-inch meatballs. Should make approximately 24 meatballs. Bake for 25 minutes. Blot well with your paper towel.

4. Bring a large skillet of water to a boil. Cook spaghetti in for 8 to 10 minutes until tender. Drain and move to your serving bowl.

5. Meanwhile, bring your sauce to a simmer in a Dutch oven. Add your meatballs to the sauce and simmer, for 20 minutes, while covered. Stir in your parsley.

6. Top your spaghetti with your sauce and meatballs. Add your grated cheese as desired.

7. Serve and Enjoy!

Mediterranean Chicken with Eggplant
Servings: 5

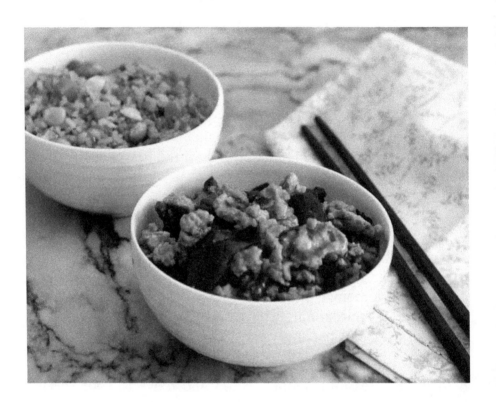

Ingredients

- 3 Peeled Eggplants (Cut Lengthwise Into 1/2 Inch Thick Slices)
- 6 Diced Skinless Boneless Chicken Breast Halves
- 3 tablespoons of Olive Oil Diced Onion
- 1/2 cup of Water tablespoons of Tomato Paste
- 2 teaspoons of Dried Oregano
- Pepper
- Salt

Directions:

1.   Place your eggplant strips in a large skillet of lightly salted water and allow to soak for approximately 30 minutes.

2.   Remove eggplant from your skillet and lightly brush with olive oil. Saute eggplant until lightly browned. Place in a 9x13 inch baking dish. Set to the side.

3.   Saute your onion and diced chicken in a large sized skillet over a medium heat. Stir in your water and tomato paste. Cover the skillet and reduce the heat to low. Allow to simmer for approximately 10 minutes.

4.   Preheat your oven to 400 degrees. Pour your chicken / tomato mixture over the eggplant. Season with salt, pepper, and oregano. Cover with aluminum foil. Bake for approximately 20 minutes.

5.   Serve and Enjoy!

Spicy Mediterranean Chicken with Sausage-Stuffed Cherry Peppers
Servings: 6

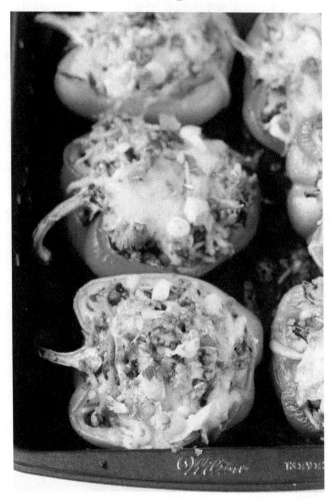

Ingredients

- 18 Cherry Peppers (In Brine)
- 2 tablespoons of Ground Cumin
- 1 Teaspoon of Salt
- 6 ounces of Fresh Italian Sausage
- 1 Sliced Onion

- Tablespoons of Olive Oil Cloves of Crushed Garlic
- 1/2 teaspoon of Crushed Red Pepper Flakes
- 1 tablespoon of Herbes De Provence
- 1 cup of Sliced Pepperoncini Peppers w/ Juices
- 2 cups of Chicken Stock
- 1 tablespoon of Ground Black Pepper
- 14-ounce can of Artichoke Hearts (Drained & Chopped)
- 1 tablespoon of Chopped Fresh Basil
- 1/2 cup of Pitted Kalamata Olives
- 1 tablespoon of Chopped Fresh Marjoram
- 1 tablespoon of Chopped Fresh Oregano

Directions:

1.   Preheat your oven to 350 degrees.

2.   Place your chicken thighs in a big bowl. Season with cumin, salt, and black pepper. Set to the side.

3.   Stuff each of your cherry peppers generously with your Italian sausage. Set to the side.

4.   Heat your olive oil in a Dutch oven over a medium-high heat. Place your chicken thighs, facing skin-side down, in your pan and cook for about 5 minutes until brown. Turn the chicken over and brown the other side for about 1 minute. Remove your chicken from the pan.

5.   Cook your onion in the Dutch oven over a medium-high heat. Cook and stir for approximately 5 minutes until the onion has caramelized. Reduce your heat to medium and stir in the herbes de Provence, garlic, and crushed red pepper.

6.   Stir in the pepperoncini and its juices. Cook for 2 minutes until warmed through. Remove from the heat.

7.   Place your chicken, skin-side up, in a single layer over top your onions and pepperoncini in the Dutch oven. Pour your stock into the pan until it is nearly covering the chicken.

8.   Sprinkle your olives, artichoke hearts, and stuffed cherry peppers over top of the chicken.

9.   Return to a medium-high heat and bring it to a simmer.

10.   Cover and roast in your preheated oven for approximately 1 hour until the sausage is cooked through and the liquid is bubbling.

11.   Garnish with your oregano, chopped basil, and marjoram

12.   Serve and Enjoy!

Moussaka
Servings: 6

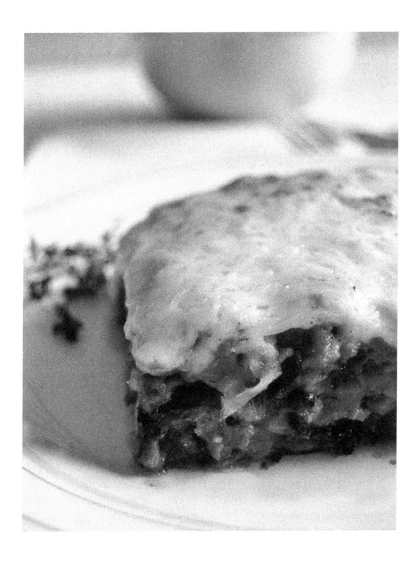

Ingredients

- 2 pound of Ground Turkey

- 1 teaspoon of Ground Cinnamon cups of Plain Nonfat Yogurt
- 1 Yellow Onion (Cut into 1/4-Inch Dice)
- 28-ounce can of Whole Peeled Tomatoes (Chopped Coarsely)
- 1/4 teaspoon of Ground Nutmeg
- 1 clove of Minced Garlic Medium Eggplants
- 1 /4 teaspoon of Ground Pepper
- 1 teaspoon of Coarse Salt
- 1/4 cup of Chopped Fresh Oregano
- 1/4 cup of Tomato Paste
- 1/2 cup of Chopped Fresh Flat-Leaf Parsley
- 1/4 cup of Grated Parmesan Cheese
- Olive Oil

Directions:

1.   Drain your yogurt into a cheesecloth-lined sieve until it is thickened. At least 2 hours or overnight.

2.   Place your turkey in a medium-sized saucepan over a medium heat. Cook it until it is browned. Should take approximately 6 minutes. Using a slotted spoon, transfer over to a medium-sized bowl. Add your garlic, onion, salt, cinnamon, pepper, and nutmeg to your saucepan. Cook for approximately 10 minutes until the onion is translucent. Return your turkey to the saucepan with tomato paste, tomatoes, and oregano. Bring it to a boil, reduce the heat to a medium-low heat. Simmer until your sauce has thickened. Should take approximately 1 hour. Remove it from the heat. Stir in your chopped parsley. Set to the side.

3.   Preheat your broiler. While your sauce cooks, cut your eggplants into 1/4-inch slices. Sprinkle both sides with salt. Place in a colander over your bowl. Allow to stand for 1 hour to drain. Press out the water. Lay the dried slices on a baking sheet. Coat it with olive oil and broil for 2 minutes until browned. Turn the

slices and coat with olive oil. Broil for another 2 minutes until browned. Repeat until all of your slices are broiled. Set you cooked eggplant to the side.

4. Place your drained yogurt in a small-sized bowl. Add your eggs and Parmesan. Whisk together briskly. Set to the side.

5. Preheat your oven to 400 degrees. Place a layer of eggplant on the bottom of your 8x8-inch baking pan. Cover with half of your turkey sauce. Place another layer of eggplant slices on top, followed by the remaining turkey sauce. Add a final eggplant layer and cover with your yogurt mixture. Bake for 30 minutes until the top starts to brown and the mixture is bubbling. Transfer to a heat-proof surface. Allow to rest for 10 minutes until it cools and begins to get firm. Cut into squares.

6. Serve and Enjoy!

Sweet Sausage Marsala
Servings: 6

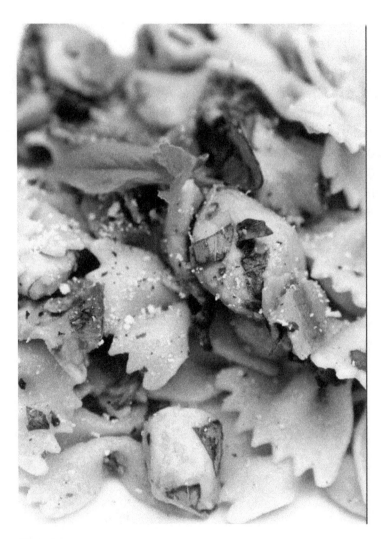

Ingredients

- 16-ounce package of Farfalle Pasta
- 1 Pound of Mild Italian Sausage Links
- 1 clove of Minced Garlic

- 1 Sliced Medium Green Bell Pepper
- 1/2 of Sliced Large Onion
- 1/3 cup of Water
- 1 tablespoon of Marsala Wine
- 1 Sliced Medium Red Bell Pepper
- 14.5-ounce can of Italian Style Diced Tomatoes
- Pinch of Black Pepper
- Pinch of Dried Oregano

Directions:

1. Bring a skillet of water to a boil. Cook your pasta until al dente. Should take approximately 8 to 10 minutes. Drain pasta.

2. Place your sausages and 1/3 cup of water in a skillet over a medium-high heat. Cover and cook for 5 to 8 minutes. Drain and slice thinly.

3. Return your sausage to the skillet. Stir in your onions, garlic, Marsala wine, and peppers. Cook over a medium-high heat. Stir frequently until the sausage is cooked through. Stir in your black pepper, diced tomatoes, and oregano. Cook another 2 minutes. Remove from heat. Add over top your cooked pasta.

4. Serve and Enjoy!

Shrimps Saganaki
Servings: 4

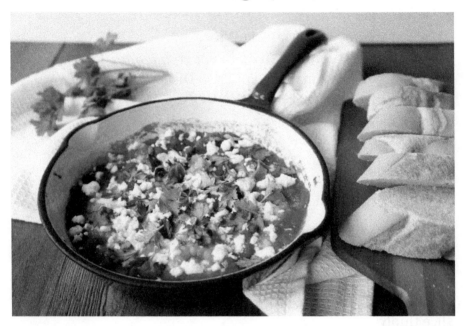

Ingredients

- Pound of Medium Shrimps w/ Shells
- 1 Chopped Onion
- 1 cup of White Wine
- Tablespoons of Chopped Fresh Parsley
- 14.5-ounce can of Diced Tomatoes
- 1/4 cup of Olive Oil
- 8-   ounce package of Feta Cheese Cubed
- Salt
- Pepper
- 1/4 teaspoon of Garlic Powder

Directions:

1.   Bring 2 inches of water to a boil in your large saucepan. Add your shrimp, the water should barely cover them. Boil for approximately 5 minutes. Drain and reserve the liquid. Set to the side.

2.   Heat 2 tablespoons of your oil in a saucepan. Add your onions. Cook until the onions are soft. Mix in your wine, parsley, garlic powder, tomatoes, and remaining olive oil. Simmer for approximately 30 minutes, stirring occasionally until the sauce has thickened.

3.   While your sauce is simmering, remove the legs of the shrimp and pull off the shells, leaving the head and tail. You can remove the legs by pinching them.

4.   Once the sauce has thickened, stir in your shrimp and shrimp stock. Bring to a simmer and cook for approximately 5 minutes. Add your feta cheese and remove it from the heat. Allow to stand until the cheese begins to melt.

5.   Serve and Enjoy!

Simple Mediterranean Fish
Servings: 4

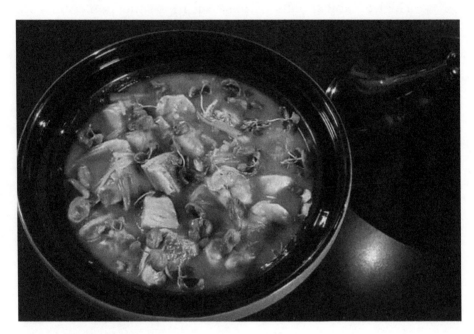

Ingredients

- 4 6-ounce Halibut Fillets Chopped Onion
- 1 Large Chopped Tomato
- 5-ounce jar of Pitted Kalamata Olives
- 1 tablespoon of Greek Seasoning
- 1 tablespoon of Lemon Juice
- 1/4 cup of Olive Oil
- 1/4 cup of Capers
- Pepper Salt

Directions:

1.   Preheat your oven to 350 degrees.

2.   Place your halibut fillets on a sheet of aluminum foil and season using your Greek seasoning.

3.   Combine your tomato, olives, onion, capers, lemon juice, olive oil, pepper, and salt in a bowl. Spoon your mixture over the halibut. Carefully seal the edges of your aluminum foil to create a packet. Place the packet on your baking sheet.

4.   Bake for 30 to 40 minutes until the fish flakes easily with a fork.

5.   Serve and Enjoy!

Mussels Marinara di Amore
Servings: 4

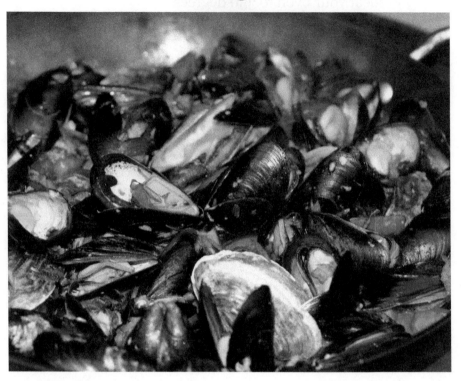

Ingredients

- 8 ounces of Linguini Pasta
- pound of Mussels (Cleaned & Debearded)
- 1 clove of Minced Garlic
- 1 tablespoon of Olive Oil
- 14.5-ounce can of Crushed Tomatoes
- 1/2 teaspoon of Dried Basil
- 1/2 teaspoon of Dried Oregano
- 1/4 cup of White Wine
- Pinch of Crushed Red Pepper Flakes
- 1 Lemon (Cut Into Wedges)

Directions:

1.   In a large sized skillet over a medium heat, warm your oil and saute your garlic until it is transparent.

2.   Add your oregano, tomato, red pepper flakes, and basil to the skillet. Reduce the heat to low and simmer for approximately 5 minutes.

3.   Add your mussels and wine to the skillet. Cover and increase the heat to high for approximately 3 to 5 minutes until the mussel shells have opened.

4.   Pour mussels mixture over your pasta and sprinkle with parsley. Squeeze your lemon wedges over top of it. Garnish with remaining lemon.

5.   Serve and Enjoy!

Curry Salmon with Napa Slaw
Servings: 4

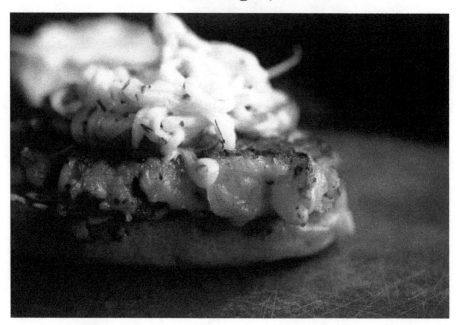

Ingredients

- 4 6-ounce Salmon Fillets cup of Brown Basmati Rice
- tablespoons of Grape Seed Oil
- 3 teaspoons of Curry Powder
- pound of Thinly Sliced Napa Cabbage
- 1/2 cup of Fresh Mint Leaves
- 1 pound of Grated Carrots
- 1/4 cup of Lime Juice
- Coarse Salt Ground Pepper

Directions:

1.   In a saucepan, bring 2 cups of water to a boil. Add your rice and season with pepper and salt. Cover saucepan and reduce heat

to a medium-low. Cook approximately 30 to 35 minutes until tender.

2.   In a big bowl, combine your carrots, cabbage, lime juice, mint, and oil. Season with pepper and salt. Toss to combine.

3.   Heat your broiler and set rack 4 inches from the heat. Approximately 10 minutes before rice is finished cooking, place your salmon on a baking sheet lined with foil. Rub your salmon with curry. Season with pepper, and salt. Broil for 6 to 8 minutes until cooked through.

4.   Fluff rice with a fork and add it alongside your salad and fish.

5.   Serve and Enjoy!

Greek Fava with Grilled Squid
Servings: 6

- 12 ounces of Squid (Cleaned)
- 3 tablespoons of Extra-Virgin Olive Oil 2 cups of Vegetable Broth
- Small Finely Chopped Red Onion 3/4 cup of Yellow Split Peas tablespoons of Lemon Juice
- 1/4 teaspoon of Ground Pepper 3/4 teaspoon of Salt
- tablespoons of Finely Chopped Fresh Parsley Lemon (Cut Into Wedges)
- Skewers

Directions:

1.   Rinse your split peas under some running water to remove any pebbles or grit.

2.   Heat 1 tablespoon of oil over a medium heat in a large-sized saucepan. Add your onion and cook for approximately 5 minutes until softened. Add your split peas and toss to coat. Add your broth and bring to a boil over a high heat. Reduce your heat to a simmer and cover. Cook for 45 minutes to 1 hour, stirring occasionally and skimming any foam off the surface. Split peas should be tender and most of the liquid should be absorbed. If the liquid is gone before the peas are finished add a little more liquid and continue to cook.

3.   Cut the body of your squid into 1/2-inch rings, leave the tentacles whole. Combine the tentacles and rings with 1/2 teaspoon of salt, 1 1/2 teaspoons of oil, and 1/4 teaspoon of pepper in a medium-sized bowl. Set to the side.

4.   Transfer your peas to a food processor. Add lemon juice, 1 1/2 teaspoons of oil, and the last 1/4 teaspoon of salt. Process your mixture until creamy, with the consistency of mashed potatoes. Spread this mixture onto your serving platter.

5.   Preheat your grill to a medium-high heat. Thread your tentacles and squid rings on skewers. Oil your grill rack. Grill your squid, turning once until tender but firm. Should take about 4 minutes in total.

6.   Remove the squid from the skewers and arrange on top of your fava mixture. Drizzle remaining 1 tablespoon of oil on top. Season with pepper and sprinkle with parsley. Add lemon wedges to the side.

7.   Serve and Enjoy!

Salmon Panzanella
Servings: 4

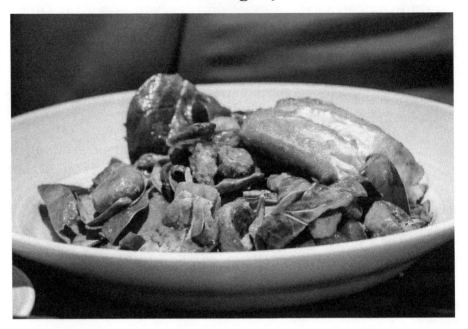

Ingredients

- pound of Center Cut Salmon (Skinned & Cut Into 4 Portions)
- 8 Pitted & Chopped Kalamata Olives
- tablespoons of Extra-Virgin Olive Oil
- 1 tablespoon of Chopped Capers
- Large Tomatoes (Cut Into 1-Inch Pieces)
- 2 slices of Thick Day Old Whole Grain Bread (Cut Into 1-Inch Cubes)
- tablespoons of Red Wine Vinegar
- 1 Medium Peeled Cucumber (Cut Into 1-Inch Cubes)
- 1/4 cup of Thinly Sliced Fresh Basil
- 1/4 cup of Thinly Sliced Red Onion
- 1/2 teaspoon of Kosher Salt

Directions:

1. Preheat your grill to high.

2. Whisk your vinegar, capers, olives, and 1/8 teaspoon of pepper in a big bowl. Slowly whisk in your oil until well combined. Add your tomatoes, bread, onion, cucumber, and basil.

3. Grill the salmon until it is cooked through. Should take 4 to 5 minutes per side.

4. Divide your salad among 4 separate plates and top each one with a piece of your salmon.

5. Serve and Enjoy!

Tilapia Feta Florentine
Servings: 4

Ingredients

- 1 pound of Tilapia Fillets
- 1/4 cup of Chopped Onion teaspoons of Olive Oil
- clove of Minced Garlic
- 1/4 cup of Kalamata Olives
- 9-ounce bags of Fresh Spinach
- tablespoons of Crumbled Feta Cheese
- 1/2 teaspoon of Salt
- 1/2 teaspoon of Grated Lemon Rind
- 1/8 teaspoon of White Pepper
- teaspoons of Lemon Juice
- 1/4 teaspoon of Dried Oregano
- 2 tablespoons of Melted Butter
- 1 Pinch of Paprika

Directions:

1.   Preheat your oven to 400 degrees.

2.   Heat your olive oil over a medium heat in a large sized skillet. Cook and stir your garlic and onion for approximately 5 minutes until the onion is soft. Add your spinach and cook for 5 minutes until the spinach has wilted and cooked down. Stir in your feta cheese, olives, salt, lemon rind, white pepper, and oregano. Continue to cook until the cheese has all melted and the flavors are blended. Should take another 5 minutes.

3.   Spread your spinach mixture into a 9x13 inch baking dish. Arrange your fillets over the spinach mixture. Mix together your

lemon juice and butter in a small sized bowl and drizzle over your fish. Sprinkle with a pinch of paprika.

4.   Bake your fish approximately 20 to 25 minutes until the flesh has turned opaque and flakes easily.

5.   Serve and Enjoy!

Seafood Couscous Paella
Servings: 4

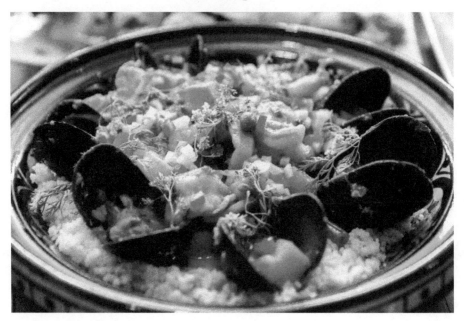

Ingredients

- 4 ounces of Peeled & Deveined Small Shrimp
- 4 ounces of Bay Scallops (Tough Muscle Removed)
- 1/2 cup of Whole-Wheat Couscous
- 2 teaspoons of Extra-Virgin Olive Oil
- 1 Clove of Minced Garlic
- 1 Medium Chopped Onion
- 1/2 teaspoon of Fennel Seed
- 1/2 teaspoon of Dried Thyme
- 1/4 teaspoon of Ground Pepper
- 1/4 teaspoon of Salt
- 1/4 cup of Vegetable Broth
- 1 cup of Canned Diced Tomatoes (No Salt Added w/ Juice)
- Pinch of Crumbled Saffron Threads

Directions:

1.   Heat your oil in a saucepan over a medium heat. Add your onion and cook for 3 minutes, stirring constantly. Add your thyme, garlic, pepper, salt, fennel seed, and saffron. Cook approximately 20 seconds.

2.   Stir in your broth and tomatoes. Bring to a simmer. Cover and reduce the heat. Simmer for approximately 2 minutes.

3.   Increase your heat to medium, stir in your scallops and cook for 2 minutes, stirring occasionally. Add your shrimp and cook for 2 more minutes. Stir in your couscous. Cover and remove from the heat. Allow to stand for 5 minutes. Fluff.

4.   Serve and Enjoy!

Lemon-Garlic Marinated Shrimp
Servings: 12

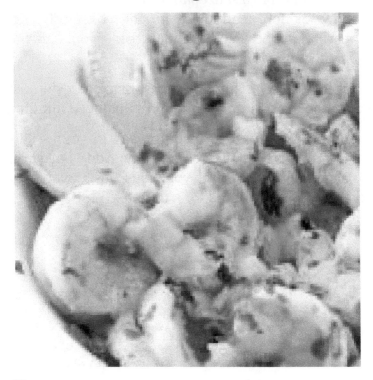

Ingredients

- 1/4 pounds of Cooked Shrimp
- 2 Tablespoons of Extra-Virgin Olive Oil
- 2 Tablespoons of Minced Garlic
- 1/4 cup of Lemon Juice
- 1/2 teaspoon of Kosher Salt
- 1/4 cup of Minced Fresh Parsley
- 1/2 teaspoon of Pepper

Directions:

1.   Place your garlic and oil in a small-sized skillet and cook over a medium heat for 1 minute until fragrant. Add your parsley,

lemon juice, pepper and salt. Toss with your shrimp in a large bowl. Chill until ready to serve.

2.	Serve and Enjoy!

Mustard Trout and Lady Apples
Servings: 4

Ingredients

- 8 3-ounce Trout Fillets
- 4 Lady Apples (Cut In Half) Minced Shallot
- Tablespoons of Extra-Virgin Olive Oil
- Tablespoons of Fine Plain Bread Crumbs
- 1 teaspoon of Chopped Fresh Thyme
- tablespoon of Melted Unsalted Butter 1 cup of Apple Cider
- teaspoons of Light Brown Sugar 1 tablespoon of Rinsed Capers
- 1 tablespoon of Dijon Mustard
- Pepper Coarse Salt

Directions:

1.   Preheat your oven to 375 degrees. In a little bowl, combine your thyme, breadcrumbs, and shallot. Season with pepper and salt. Add your butter and toss well to combine.

2.   Place all your apples cut-side up in a large baking dish. Sprinkle with sugar and top with your bread crumb mixture. Pour 1/4 cup of cider around the apples. Cover and bake approximately 30 minutes. Uncover and bake for 20 minutes more until the apples are tender and the crumbs are crispy. Remove it from the oven.

3.   Turn oven to a broil and place your rack 4 inches from the heat source. Pat your trout fillets dry. Season each side with pepper and salt. Brush your baking sheet with 1 tablespoon of oil. Place your trout skin-side up on your baking sheet. Brush your trout skin with the remaining 1 tablespoon of oil. Broil for 6

minutes until the trout is cooked through. Reheat your apples on the shelf directly underneath the trout so your crumbs don't burn for the last 1 to 2 minutes.

4.   In a small-sized saucepan, whisk 3/4 cup of cider, capers, and mustard until combined. Cook over a medium-high heat for 5 to 7 minutes until reduced to a sauce consistency. Place two trout fillets side by side on each of your four plates. Spoon the juices around the fish, Set the two apple halves next to each of fillets.

5.   Serve and Enjoy!

Grilled Sardines over Wilted Baby Arugula
Servings: 4

Ingredients

- 16 Fresh Sardines (Innards & Gills Removed)
- 2 teaspoons of Extra-Virgin Olive Oil
- 2 Large Bunches of Trimmed Baby Arugula
- Ground Pepper
- Kosher Salt
- Lemon Wedges (For Garnish)

Directions:

1.   Prepare your grill or griddle. Rinse your arugula, shaking off the excess water. Arrange on your platter and set to the side.

2.   Rinse your sardines in cold water, rubbing them to remove the scales. Wipe them dry. In your bowl, combine the olive oil and sardines. Toss well to coat.

3.   Grill the sardines over a high heat or hot coals for approximately 2 to 3 minutes per side. Sardines are done once they are golden and crispy. Season with pepper and salt. Transfer them to your arugula-lined platter and add lemon wedges as garnish.

4.   Serve and Enjoy!

Flounder Mediterranean
Servings: 4

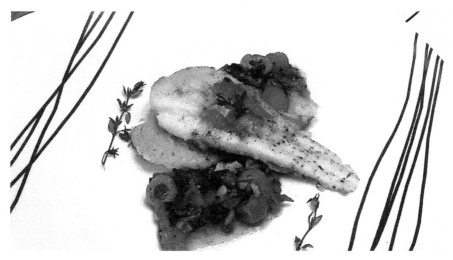

Ingredients

- Pound of Flounder Fillets 5 Roma Tomatoes
- 1/2 of a Spanish Onion
- Tablespoons of Extra-Virgin Olive Oil
- Cloves of Chopped Garlic
- 24 Pitted & Chopped Kalamata Olives
- Tablespoons of Freshly Grated Parmesan Cheese
- 1/4 cup of Capers
- 1/4 cup of White Wine Teaspoon of Fresh Lemon Juice
- Leaves of Fresh Basil (Torn)
- Leaves of Fresh Basil (Chopped)
- Pinch of Italian Seasoning

Directions:

1.   Preheat your oven to 425 degrees.

2.   Bring a saucepan of water to a boil. Put your tomatoes into the boiling water and immediately remove to a bowl of ice water. Drain water. Remove and discard the skins from the tomatoes. Chop the tomatoes and set to the side.

3.   Heat your olive oil over a medium heat in a skillet. Saute your onion for approximately 5 minutes until tender. Stir in your garlic, tomatoes, and Italian seasoning. Cook for 5 to 7 minutes until the tomatoes are tender. Mix in your wine, olives, lemon juice, capers, and chopped basil. Reduce the heat, blend in your Parmesan cheese, and cook until your mixture is reduced to a thick sauce. Should take approximately 15 minutes.

4.   Place your flounder in a shallow baking dish. Pour your sauce over the fillets and top with the torn basil leaves.

5.   Bake for approximately 12 minutes. Once finished, the fish should be easily flaked using your fork.

6.   Serve and Enjoy!

Spanish Cod
Servings: 6

Ingredients

- 6 4-ounce Cod Fillets Tablespoon of Olive Oil
- 1 tablespoon of Butter
- Tablespoons of Chopped Fresh Garlic
- 1/4 cup of Finely Chopped Onion
- 15 Cherry Tomatoes (Halved)
- 1 cup of Tomato Sauce
- 1/2 cup of Chopped Green Olives
- 1/4 cup of Deli Marinated Italian Vegetable Salad (Coarsely Chopped)
- Dash of Cayenne Pepper
- Dash of Black Pepper
- Dash of Paprika

Directions:

1. Heat your olive oil and butter over a medium heat in a large skillet. Cook garlic and onions until slightly tender. Stir occasionally. Don't burn the garlic. Add your cherry tomatoes and tomato sauce. Bring to a simmer. Stir in your marinated vegetable salad and green olives. Season with cayenne pepper, black pepper, and paprika.

2. Cook your fillets for 5 to 8 minutes in the sauce over a medium heat.

3. Serve and Enjoy!

Mediterranean Pasta with Basil
Servings: 4

Ingredients:

- 350 g dried pasta (whole-wheat corkscrew)
- 3 garlic cloves, coarsely chopped
- 2 tablespoons olive oil, plus more to serve
- 2 red peppers, seeded, cut into chunks
- 2 red onions, cut into wedges
- 2 mild red chili, seeded, diced
- Teaspoon golden caster sugar
- 1 kg small ripe tomatoes, quartered
- Tablespoon grated Parmesan, to serve
- 1 handful fresh basil leaves, to serve

Directions:

To roast the vegetables:

1.   Preheat gas oven to 200C, gas to 6, or fan to 180C.

2.   Scatter the peppers, the red peppers, the chilies, and the garlic into a large-sized roasting tin.

3.   Sprinkle with the sugar and then drizzle with the olive oil; season well with the salt and the pepper.

4.   Roast for about 15 minutes. Toss the tomatoes in the tin and then roast for additional 15 minutes, or until the vegetables are soft and golden.

For the pasta:

5.   While the vegetables are roasting, cook the pasta according to the instructions of the package until tender with still a little bit of bite; drain well.

6.   Remove the roasted vegetables from oven. Add the pasta into the tin; toss lightly to mix.

7.   Tear the basil leaves and sprinkle over the pasta mixture. Sprinkle with the parmesan cheese.

8.   Buon Appettito!

Lemon Curd Filled Almond-Lemon Cake

Servings: 8

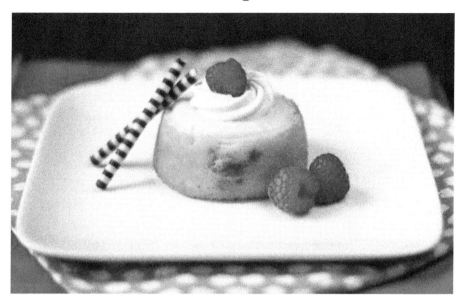

Ingredients

- 4 large egg yolks
- 4 large egg whites
- 2 teaspoons matzo cake meal
- 2 cups fresh raspberries
- 1/4 teaspoon of salt
- 1/4 cup matzo cake meal
- 1/4 cup blanched almonds, ground
- 1/2 teaspoon grated lemon rind
- teaspoon lemon juice, fresh
- 1 cup sugar
- 1 cup Lemon Curd
- 1 1/2 teaspoons water
- Cooking spray

Directions:

1.   Preheat the oven to 350F.

2.   Coat a 9-inch spring-form pan with the cooking spray. Dust the pan with the 2 teaspoons of matzo cake meal.

3.   Place the yolks into a large-sized bowl; beat with a mixer at high speed for about 2 minutes. Gradually add the sugar and beat the mixture until pale and thick, about 1 minute. Add the 1/4 cup matzo cake meal, water, lemon rind, lemon juice, and salt; beat until the mixture is just blended. Fold in the almonds.

4.   Bake for about 35 minutes at 350F or until the cake is set and brown; remove the pan from the oven, place in a wire rack, and let cool for 10 minutes. Run a knife around the edge of the cake, remove the cake from the pan, place in the wire rack and let cool completely. The cake will sink as it cools.

5.   Spread about 1 cup of lemon curd in the center of the cake. Top with the raspberries. Cut the cake into 8 wedges with a serrated knife. Serve immediately.

Greek Almond Rounds Shortbread
Servings: 20

Ingredients

- 1/2 cups butter, softened
- cup blanched almonds, lightly toasted and finely ground
- cup powdered sugar
- egg yolks
- tablespoons brandy or orange juice
- tablespoons rose flower water, (optional)
- teaspoons vanilla
- 1/2 cups cake flour
- Powdered sugar

Directions:

1. Using an electric mixer, beat the butter on MEDIUM or HIGH speed for about 30 seconds in a large sized bowl. Add the 1 cup powdered sugar; beat until the mixture is light in color and fluffy, occasionally scraping the bowl as needed.

2. Beat in the yolks, vanilla, and the brandy until combined.

3. With a wooden spoon, stir in the flour and almonds until well incorporated. Cover and refrigerate for about 1 hour or until chilled and the dough is easy to handle.

4. Preheat the oven to 325F.

5. Place the cookie sheet into the preheated oven; bake for about 12-14 minutes or until the cookies are set.

6. When the cookies are baked, transfer them on wire racks. While they are still warm, brush with the rose water, if desired.

Sprinkle with more powdered sugar. Let cool completely on the wire racks.

Frozen Mediterranean Delight
Servings: 4

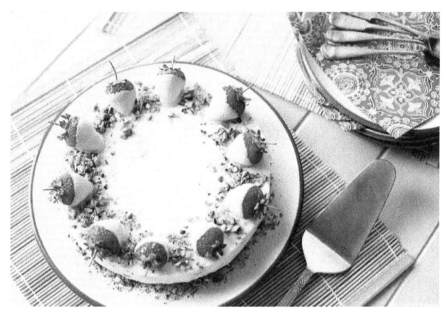

Ingredients

- 6 pitted dates, chopped
- 3 cups yogurt, plain, nonfat
- 2/3 cup pistachios, natural, unsalted, shelled
- 2 ounces bittersweet chocolate
- 1/2 cup sugar tablespoon ouzo

Directions:

1.   Line a fine meshed strainer with cheesecloth. Place the strainer over a bowl. Put the yogurt in the cheesecloth lines strainer; allow to drain for 2 hours.

2.   Put the sugar and half of the pistachios in a coffee grinder or a food processor, grind or process until powder.

3.   Roughly chop the remaining pistachios.

4.   Combine the drained yogurt, nuts, sugar-pistachio mixture, ouzo, and dates, mixing until well incorporated; place in the freezer. After 1 hour, remove from the freezer and mix well. Return to the freezer and freeze until firm.

5.   Divide into 4 servings. Garnish with chocolate shavings; serve.

Slow Cooker Rosemary and Red Pepper Chicken

Servings: 8

Ingredients

- Medium Thinly Sliced Red Bell Pepper (Seeded)
- 1 Small Thinly Sliced Onion
- 4 cloves of Minced Garlic
- 1/2 teaspoon of Dried Oregano teaspoons of Dried Rosemary
- 8 ounces of Turkey Italian Sausages (Casings Removed)
- 8 4-ounce Skinless Boneless Chicken Breast Halves
- 1/4 cup of Dry Vermouth
- 1/4 teaspoon of Coarsely Ground Pepper 1 1/2 tablespoons of Cornstarch
- 1/4 cup of Chopped Fresh Parsley tablespoons of Cold Water
- Salt

Directions:

1.   In a 6-quart slow cooker, combine your onion, garlic, bell pepper, oregano, and rosemary. Crumble your sausages over the onion mixture.

2.   Rinse your chicken and pat it dry. Arrange in a single layer over your sausage. Sprinkle with your pepper. Pour in your

vermouth. Cover and cook for 5 to 7 hours on the low setting. Chicken should be tender and cooked through when done.

3.   Transfer your chicken to a warm platter and cover to keep it warm.

4.   In a bowl, stir together your cold water and cornstarch. Stir the cooking liquid in your slow cooker. Increase the heat to high and cover. Cook, stirring a few times until the sauce has thickened. Should take about 10 minutes. Season with salt. Spoon your sauce over the chicken and sprinkle with parsley.

5.   Serve and Enjoy!

Greek Penne and Chicken

Servings: 4

Ingredients

- 16-ounce package of Penne Pasta
- pound of Skinless Boneless Chicken Breast Halves (Cut Into Bite Sized Pieces)
- 1/2 cup of Chopped Red Onion 1 1/2 tablespoons of Butter cloves of Minced Garlic
- 14-ounce can of Artichoke Hearts 1 Chopped Tomato
- tablespoons of Chopped Fresh Parsley 1/2 cup of Crumbled Feta Cheese
- 2 tablespoons of Lemon Juice
- teaspoon of Dried Oregano Ground Black Pepper
- Salt

Directions:

1. In a large sized skillet over a medium-high heat, melt your butter. Add your garlic and onion. Cook approximately 2 minutes. Add your chopped chicken and continue to cook until golden brown. Should take approximately 5 to 6 minutes. Stir occasionally.

2. Reduce your heat to a medium-low. Drain and chop your artichoke hearts. Add them to your skillet along with your chopped tomato, fresh parsley, feta cheese, dried oregano, lemon juice, and drained pasta. Cook for 2 to 3 minutes until heated through.

3. Season with your ground black pepper and salt.

4. Serve and Enjoy!

Herbed Lamb Chops w/ Greek Couscous Salad

Servings: 4

Ingredients

- 2   1/2 pounds of Lamb Loin Chops (Trim The Fat Off)
- 1/2 cup of Whole-Wheat Couscous
- tablespoon of Minced Garlic cup of Water
- 1/4 teaspoon of Salt
- 1 tablespoon of Finely Chopped Fresh Parsley
- Medium Chopped Tomatoes
- teaspoons of Extra-Virgin Olive Oil
- 1 Medium Peeled & Chopped Cucumber tablespoons of Lemon Juice
- 1/2 cup of Crumbled Feta
- tablespoons of Finely Chopped Fresh Dill

Directions:

1.   Bring water to a boil in a medium-sized saucepan.

2.   Combine your parsley, salt, and garlic in a small-sized bowl.

Press your garlic mixture into each side of the lamb chops. Heat oil over a medium-high heat in a large skillet. Add your lamb chops and cook approximately 5 to 6 minutes per side until you've reached the desired level of cooked. Keep them warm until it is time to serve.

3.   Stir your couscous into your boiling water. Return to a boil, reduce heat to a low simmer, cover and cook approximately 2 minutes. Remove from the heat and allow to stand uncovered for 5 minutes. Fluff couscous with your fork. Transfer over to a medium bowl. Add your cucumber, tomatoes, lemon juice, dill, and feta. Stir well to combine.

4.   Serve and Enjoy!

Sicilian Lemon Chicken w/ Raisin-Tomato Sauce

Servings: 4

Ingredients

- 4 6-ounce Skinless Boneless Chicken Breast Halves
- 4 tablespoons of Extra-Virgin Olive Oil
- 16-ounce package of Angel Hair Pasta
- 3/4 cup of Golden Raisins
- 4 sprigs of Fresh Basil Lemon (Juiced & Zested)
- 1 Medium Thinly Sliced Onion
- 1/4 cup of Shaved Parmesan Cheese
- 1/4 teaspoon of Cayenne Pepper
- tablespoon of Minced Garlic
- tablespoons of Chopped Black Olives tablespoons of Pine Nuts
- Bay Leaves
- 15-ounce can of Diced Tomatoes (Drained)
- 1/4 teaspoon of Dried Oregano
- tablespoon of Balsamic Vinegar
- tablespoons of Julienned Fresh Basil
- 1 teaspoon of White Sugar
- Pepper
- Salt

Directions:

1.   Soak your raisins in warm water for 10 minutes until plump. Drain and set to the side.

2.   Heat 3 tablespoons of your olive oil over a medium-high heat in a saucepan. Stir in your garlic, onion, olives, and pine nuts. Season with oregano, cayenne, and bay leaves. Cook for 5 minutes until the onions have softened. Stir in your tomatoes and season with pepper and salt. Cook for another 5 minutes. Add your balsamic vinegar, raisins, and sugar. Cook approximately 5 minutes until thickened. Remove your bay leaves and stir in your basil. Cover and keep warm.

3.   Bring a skillet of water to a boil. Cook your pasta for 8 to 10 minutes until al dente. Drain.

4.   Heat 1 tablespoon of olive oil over a medium heat in a skillet. Toss your chicken with lemon juice to coat. Cook chicken on both sides until cooked through. Should take approximately 15 minutes. Transfer to a warm plate and let rest for 5 minutes.

5.   Serve and Enjoy!

Braised Chicken with Olives

Servings: 4

Ingredients

- 4 Whole Chicken Legs (Skinned & Cut Into Drumsticks & Thighs)
- tablespoon of Olive Oil
- 1 Medium Diced Yellow Onion cloves of Minced Garlic
- Diced Carrots
- 1 cup of Low-Sodium Canned Chicken Broth
- 2 tablespoons of Chopped Fresh Ginger
- 1 cup of Dry White Wine
- 1 cup of Water
- 1/2 cup of Pitted & Chopped Green Olives
- 1/3 cup of Raisins
- 3/4 cup of Canned Chickpeas (Drained & Rinsed) sprigs of Thyme

Directions:

1.   Preheat your oven to 350 degrees.

2.   In a large skillet or Dutch oven, heat your olive oil over a medium heat. Place your chicken pieces in the skillet, being sure not to overcrowd your pan. Saute your chicken until it is nicely crisped and browned on each side. Should take about 5 minutes per side. Transfer your chicken to a big plate and set to the side.

3.   Reduce your heat to a medium-low. Add your carrots, onion, ginger, and garlic. Saute, stirring frequently until your onion is translucent and soft. Should take approximately 5

minutes. Add your chicken broth, the water, and wine. Bring to a boil and deglaze pan by scraping up any browned bits. Return your chicken to the skillet and add your thyme. Bring the liquid back to a boil; cover and transfer it to your oven. Braise for approximately 45 minutes.

4. Remove your skillet from the oven. Stir in your chickpeas, olives, and raisins. Return skillet to the oven and continue braising, uncovered, for another 20 minutes. Remove skillet from the oven and discard the thyme.

5. Serve and Enjoy!

Greek Chicken Pasta

Servings: 6

Ingredients

Directions:

pound of Skinless Chicken Breast (Cut Into Bite Sized Pieces) 16-ounce package of Linguine Pasta

cloves of Crushed Garlic

1/2 cup of Chopped Red Onion 1 tablespoon of Olive Oil

1/2 cup of Crumbled Feta Cheese

14-ounce can of Marinated Artichoke Hearts (Chopped & Drained)

1   Large Chopped Tomato tablespoons of Lemon Juice

tablespoons of Chopped Fresh Parsley 2 teaspoons of Dried Oregano

Salt Pepper

2   Lemons (Cut Into Wedges)

1.   Bring a big skillet of lightly salted water to a boil. Cook your pasta in the boiling water for approximately 8 to 10 minutes until tender. Drain pasta once cooked.

2.   Heat your olive oil over a medium-high heat in a large sized skillet. Add your garlic and onion. Saute for about 2 minutes

until fragrant. Stir in your chicken and cook until the chicken is no longer pink in the center. Should take approximately 5 to 6 minutes.

3.   Reduce your heat to a medium-low. Add your tomato, artichoke hearts, feta cheese, lemon juice, parsley, cooked pasta, and oregano. Cook and stir for 2 to 3 minutes until heated through. Remove from the heat. Season with your pepper and salt. Garnish with your lemon wedges.

4.   Serve and Enjoy!

Homemade Self-Rising Whole-Wheat Flour

Servings: 1

Ingredients:

Cup (140 grams or 4 7/8 ounces) whole-wheat flour 1⁄4-1⁄2 teaspoon salt

1 1⁄4 teaspoons baking powder

Directions:

1. Combine all of the ingredients in a large-sized airtight container; shake well to combine, and then cover.

Chicken Milano

Servings: 4

Ingredients

4 Skinless Boneless Chicken Breast Halves

2 cloves of Crushed Garlic

tablespoon of Vegetable Oil

1   teaspoon of Italian-Style Seasoning

28-ounce can of Stewed Tomatoes (Drained)

1 teaspoon of Crushed Red Pepper Flakes

9-   ounce package of Frozen Green Beans Pepper

Salt

Directions:

1.   In a large sized skillet heat your vegetable oil over a medium- high heat. Add your chicken and season with Italian-style seasoning, garlic, hot pepper flakes, pepper, and salt.

2.   Saute for approximately 5 minutes, then add your tomatoes and cook for 5 more minutes. Add your green beans and stir together. Cover your skillet, reduce the heat to a medium-low and allow to simmer for about 15 to 20 minutes.

3.   Serve and Enjoy!

Greek Salmon Burgers

Servings: 4

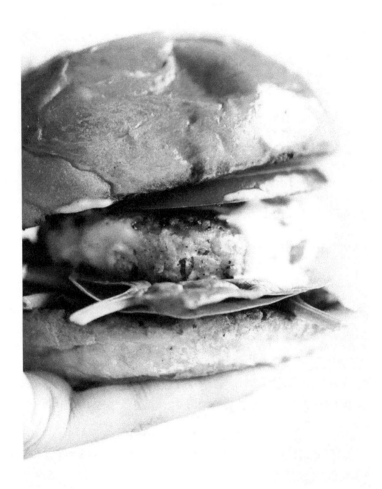

Ingredients

pound of Skinless Salmon Fillets (Cut Into 2-Inch Pieces)

1 Large Egg White

1/2 cup of Panko

1/4 teaspoon of Ground Black Pepper

1 pinch of Kosher Salt

1/2 cup of Cucumber Slices 4 Toasted Ciabatta Rolls

1/4 cup of Crumbled Feta Cheese

Directions:

1.   In your food processor, pulse your salmon, egg white, and panko until your salmon is finely chopped.

2.   Form the salmon into 4 separate patties. Each patty should be approximately 4 inches in size. Season with pepper and salt.

3.   Heat your grill to a medium-high. Cook your salmon patties, turning only once until the salmon burgers are cooked through. Should take approximately 5 to 7 minutes on each side. Toast your ciabatta rolls. Put your salmon burgers in your ciabatta rolls. Add cucumber slices on the side.

4.   Serve and Enjoy!

9 781801 457118